Say 'Good-Bye' To Belly Fat

6-Steps to Mastering Insulin and Losing Weight For Good

ISBN: 9-798410-809993 - paperback

© Copyright 2022, Sergio Rojas.
Spirit-Fueled Life

www.myforeverfatloss.com
www.get4everfit.com

Say 'Good-bye' To Belly Fat

DISCLAIMER

The material (including without limitation, advice and recommendation) within this book and any program connected to it, other programs, our email newsletter and our website is provided solely as general educational and informational purposes. Use of this program, advice and information contained herein is at the sole choice and risk of the reader.

Always consult your physician or healthcare provider before beginning any nutrition or exercise program. If you choose to use this information without prior consent of your physician, you are agreeing to accept full responsibility for your decisions and agreeing to hold harmless Sergio Rojas, Vitality by Sergio, Spirit Fueled Fitness, My Forever Fat Loss, its agents, employees, contractors and any affiliated companies from any liability with respect to injury or illness to you or your property arising out of or connected with your use of the information contained within this book, program, other programs, our email newsletter or our website.

The materials and content contained in this program, other programs, our email newsletter and our website are for general health information only and are not intended to be a substitute for professional medical advice, diagnosis or treatment. Users of this program, other programs, our email newsletter and our website should not rely exclusively on information provided in this program, other programs, our email newsletter, and our website for their own health needs. All specific medical questions should be presented to your own health care provider and you should seek medical advice before starting any type of nutrition or weight loss or workout program.

We reserve the right to update or change information contained in this book, program, other programs, our email newsletter, and our website at any time, and are not responsible for information appearing at hyperlinks.

Exercise is not without its risks and this or any other exercise program may result in injury. As with any exercise program, if at any point during your workout you begin to feel faint, dizzy or have physical discomfort, you should stop immediately and consult a medical professional. You should rely on your own review, inquiry, and assessment as to the accuracy of any information made available within.

Say 'Good-bye' To Belly Fat

"Happiness is the highest form of health." – The Dalai Lama

It's also true that when you neglect or actively damage your health, that it's a form of deep unhappiness.

I believe deeply that it is our spiritual responsibility and duty to care for and nurture our bodies and minds, so that we are able to be of service, live our higher purpose, and experience life more fully.

When you take care of your body, through nourishment, exercise, and rest, the mind will follow and also become more healthy and positive– and when you take care of your mind, through learning, creativity, connection, and meditation, your Spirit will flourish.

Developing healthy habits and becoming healthy in both body and mind starts with self-love. And self-love starts with forgiveness. Be sure to check in with yourself, release any self judgements, and truly love yourself for who and where you are today. Love your past struggles as much as your successes for the struggles have made you stronger and helped you grow far more than your successes.

If you've struggled with your weight, health, consistency, motivation, or all of the above, revisit your intention, and make sure your reason and purpose for health is connected to both a deeper part of you, and to something greater than yourself.

Lastly, do not strive for perfection– instead strive for awareness. With more awareness, you will naturally veer towards health and happiness, since that is our true nature.

Wishing You Health, Blessings, & Happy Reading,

Sergio

Say 'Good-bye' To Belly Fat

ACKNOWLEDGEMENTS

I want to thank my amazing wife Krista for always being so loving and supportive, and always believing in me. My amazing kids, Raine and Gabe, that provide me endless joy and inspiration for always wanting to lead a healthy and positive life. A deep gratitude for my parents, Jaime and Coco, my siblings, Jaime, Carlos, Sandra, and Christina, and my cousin Alex, who have been so loving and supportive my entire life, and even more so during this past year. To my dear friend and business partner, Dr. Patricia Novick for her mentorship, friendship, and selflessness. To my dear friend and spiritual guide, Nita Lapinski, who has always been so loving and helpful in all areas of my life. To my past nutrition business partners, but forever friends that continue to push and inspire me, Billy and Ana Desmond, Michael Callejas, Jordan and Kristen Kemper, Joseph Arthur, and Nate Forse. To my four brothers-from-another-mother, that have been at my side for the past 30 to over 35 years, Ed, Danny, Pete, and Matt, for always encouraging me under all the jokes and laughter. And to the endless list of clients that have trusted in me to help guide them towards better health; many of whom have been mentors of mine in so many ways, especially Rick Bayless, Clare Muñana, Jim Gallagher, John Behr, John Leinweber, Jim Laughlin, Evan Schoenberg, Karmichael Reed, Brian and Catharon Miller, Brita Miller and the late great Bernie Miller. And of course to the great Creator and Spirit, the Big G...

Love & Gratitude.

Say 'Good-bye' To Belly Fat

Table Of Contents

PREFACE   1
FOOD SCIENCE & FAT LOSS MYTHS   10
MASTER YOUR INSULIN   16
Step 1: MINDFUL EATING   17
Step 2. GET GUT HEALTHY   29
Step 3: MANAGE YOUR MACROS   39
Step 4: FASTING   58
Step 5: MOVE   63
Step 6: SLEEP   71
PUTTING IT ALL INTO PRACTICE   76
OVERCOMING OBSTACLES   80

Say 'Good-bye' To Belly Fat

PREFACE

I remember waking up one morning and catching a view of myself in the mirror as I was walking towards the bathroom in my boxer briefs and no shirt. 'Holy sh%#- what the heck has happened to me? – I thought very loudly in my head. I had man-boobs, cellulite around my rib cage, giant love handles, and very little muscle definition. I was twenty-five years old, working in a restaurant, managing a local rock band, still going to college part-time in Chicago, and somehow now also twenty-five pounds overweight. I was not used to this as I started working out and was fairly fit since I was thirteen years old. In that moment, I felt like crap, looked like crap, and realized I was headed down the wrong path. I had not been exercising much over the previous three or four years and was indulging way too much with booze and late-night munchies. My head suddenly filled up with negative thoughts about my current state and about my future. The reflection I saw in the mirror gave me a deep sinking feeling, but thankfully the metaphysical smack in the head inspired me to make a change. The very next day, I joined a gym with the determination to regain some essence of my healthier and more fit self.

Fast forward several months- I had been going to the gym two to three times per week when one day I saw a sign right outside the entrance promoting a "Transformation Challenge" with a grand prize of $1,000. At first, I got very excited because I really needed the money- somehow it seemed more attractive to me than actually transforming my body and getting fit. And trust me, I needed the transformation. Several months in, yes, I was feeling stronger and seeing a little bit of results, but not much.

Say 'Good-bye' To Belly Fat

I kept seeing signs around the gym for the transformation challenge that day, and each time I did, I would come up with another reason why I didn't need to join, and how it just wasn't right for me. Then, as I was leaving the gym, a friendly personal trainer with a massive smile and who had guided me during my gym orientation, asked me if I was going to join the transformation challenge. I figured he was just trying to sell me some personal training sessions, so I politely said, "no- I don't do challenges." - whatever that means. "I don't do challenges" - Really?? I knew deep down that I was just scared of failing and didn't want to embarrass myself. Over my next few visits to the gym, he would mention the challenge to me and encourage me without ever being pushy. He even offered me a free personal training session to help develop a workout regimen that could help me get great results and possibly win the $1,000. I couldn't turn that down even though I expected a strong sales pitch at the end of the free session to buy more training sessions. He offered but didn't push. His kindness led me to sign up for the challenge, which ended up truly changing the trajectory of my life.

No, I did not win the $1,000 or even any of the other prizes, but at the end of the 90-days, I was down 22 pounds, cut my body-fat almost in half down to 12 percent, went from a 34-inch waist down to a 31, developed good muscular definition with some ab muscles showing, and I was feeling great. Besides looking and feeling fit again, which I was thrilled about, I unexpectedly noticed a huge improvement with my anger and depression that I had been struggling with in secrecy from my family and friends. Not long after, I also began to notice how there were so many other people struggling as well, with not only their physical health, but

Say 'Good-bye' To Belly Fat

their emotional health as well. People everywhere I looked seemed so unhealthy and unhappy, and I just wanted to help everyone. I wanted them to see how simply changing their diet and exercising can make such a HUGE difference. This is what sparked my interest in becoming a personal trainer and nutritionist. I wanted to help people lose weight and feel positive and happy again. A few months later after a little research, I finally applied for my first personal training certification. Here's the crazy part- by the time I was certified, which was about ten months after completing the transformation challenge, I had gained a great deal of the weight back that I lost during the fitness transformation. I was still in decent shape, but nowhere near my fitness level of where I was at the end of the transformation challenge.

Nonetheless, I started my career as a personal trainer. It took me less than eighteen months, and I became one of the top trainers in one of the top health clubs in Chicago training 35 to 40 hours per week. But what sticks out to me the most about that time in my young career is the day my boss, the Head Trainer, approached me and said that if I wanted to stay on top in this industry and have a long successful career as a trainer, I needed to lose some weight and tone up- I needed to look more the part.

Ouch! Wow did that hurt. It was a punch in the gut. I remember defending myself by saying that people relate to me more by not being extremely fit, which can be intimidating to some people, but I knew deep down inside that I was just b.s.-ing myself. I let myself get out of shape again, but this time, I was a personal trainer. I should know better. I got back to work and vowed to never let that happen again.

Say 'Good-bye' To Belly Fat

Well, over the next ten years, I can honestly tell you that I lost and gained weight at least six or seven times! Yes, even while being a personal trainer and certified nutritionist! I tried every fitness and nutrition program on the market. And they all worked— for a little while. But every single time, I somehow gained most, if not all of my weight back within six to ten months. I was confused. I had multiple advanced certifications in exercise science as well as nutrition; my career was taking off with regular fitness segments on a local news station, working with professional athletes, speaking at conferences; but somehow, I couldn't crack the code to keeping the weight off. This was even more challenging and frustrating to me because I was telling prospects and clients that I can help them lose weight, while deep down, I wasn't sure I can help them keep it off, since I wasn't able to do that for myself.

Through Divine intervention, I met a client who is a psychologist with two PhDs. Her focus was on behavior change and habits, as well as social change and Divinity, but we'll stay focused on the behavior change and habits for now. We became close friends, and she ended up becoming a mentor to me. She spent the next few years teaching me a great deal about habits and behavior change. We eventually became business partners in our corporate wellness and professional development company. Not only did she teach me about behavior change and habits, but she also connected me to several weight loss and disease management doctors and nutritionists that practiced food as medicine. What I learned from these doctors and their courses changed everything for me. That's when I learned about the ONE key factor to losing belly fat and keeping it off—

Say 'Good-bye' To Belly Fat

the silver bullet we've all been looking for! It helped me lose twenty-one pounds plus 2.5 inches off my waist more than fourteen years ago, and I've been able to keep it off ever since, while still being able to enjoy some Chicago-style pizza, chocolate, and wine- three of my all-time favorites. I felt such a relief, coupled with so much more energy and confidence. And that is what I want for you.

That silver bullet was *Mastering my INSULIN*. If you can keep your insulin levels within a specific range most of the time, you will not only lose belly fat and excess weight but also be able to keep them both off for good. Another benefit of mastering your insulin is that you will also prevent or delay the onset of many chronic diseases like diabetes, heart disease, certain cancers, and possibly even dementia.

If only this silver bullet came in a pill, the inventor would be an instant trillionaire!! Oh wait, there is a pill for it, and the inventors (BIG Pharma) are worth billions, if not trillions, but these pills don't get to the root of mastering insulin. They bypass many natural processes to focus on the symptom, which also comes with the risk of some major side effects and other illnesses or diseases. Have you ever noticed how someone who is taking one or two medications ends up taking four or five a couple of years later; then eight to ten or even more medications after a few more years? Pumping more insulin to lower blood sugars (in Type 2 diabetics) causes weight gain plus damage to the liver and pancreas, which often lead to further complications and possibly accelerate death. Mastering your insulin is part of complex metabolic processes concerning inflammation,

Say 'Good-bye' To Belly Fat

enzymes, hormones, thyroid, liver, pancreas, brain, and gut. This book is a culmination of all the science into a simple 6-step system that you can follow to begin to master your INSULIN naturally and lose fat for good.

I wrote this book because I know so many people are extremely frustrated trying to lose weight, especially belly fat, not to mention how frustrating it is when you do lose fat and it ends up coming back with vengeance. Aside from your physical health, this also impacts your emotional health by diminishing your confidence, mood, energy, sex drive, sleep, and vitality. Whatever challenges you are going through with regards to fat loss, including mental health, I want to share these key steps that I used for myself, and for thousands of clients over the past dozen plus years, including over 700 truck drivers— many of which lost 50, even 100 plus pounds, and have been able to keep it off ever since.

Sure, some have gained a few pounds back, and it's ok and even normal to fluctuate up or down a few pounds, but they have more energy, feel more youthful and confident, sleep better, and feel more positive. Many have gotten off most or all their medications. Imagine, if you can stay within 3 to 7 pounds and within 1 inch for your waistline for the rest of your life after reaching your weight loss goal- how would that make you feel?

Add on top of that the true health benefits of getting rid of excess visceral fat around your belly and organs. Many of the truck drivers I still talk to, as well as many of my other clients, have continued to lose weight even after we finished our coaching because they simply go back to the principle of mastering their insulin using this 6-step process.

Say 'Good-bye' To Belly Fat

I want you to know that if truck drivers who have to sit for fourteen hours per day, have limited time or space to exercise, and have limited food options available to them, can lose their belly fat and keep it off, then you can too! You just have to believe in yourself and take action.

Follow the 6 steps that I'll be teaching you in this book, and you will be surprised to find that it's not as hard as you think, and it's more worth it than you thought.

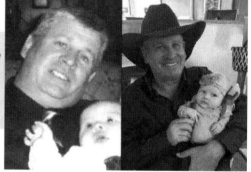

"Following Sergio's 6 Steps made it easier to lose weight than I expected. I've also gotten off all my medications, including diabetes meds, and have kept the weight off for years now."

- Roy C. Lost 82 lbs.

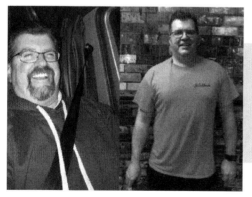

"This program has taught be to pay attention to how I feel when I eat better and exercise. You start feeling better, sleeping better, and having more energy, and it's easy to stick to what makes you feel good."

- Shawn C. Lost 45 lbs.

Say 'Good-bye' To Belly Fat

And it's not just truck drivers that have had major success using my 6-Step system to mastering insulin and losing belly fat for good.

"If they can do it, I CAN TOO!"
- You

Sergio taught me to focus on natural whole foods and pay attention to my macros. I found what worked for me was able to finally break my plateau losing over 80 pounds.

Laura K. Lost 82 pounds

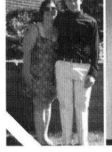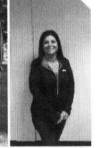

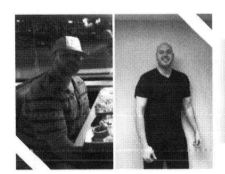

The biggest game-changer for me in Sergio's wellness program was learning Intermittent Fasting. I lost over 100 pounds and am now able to play basketball again.

Jordan E. Lost 104 lbs

Say 'Good-bye' To Belly Fat

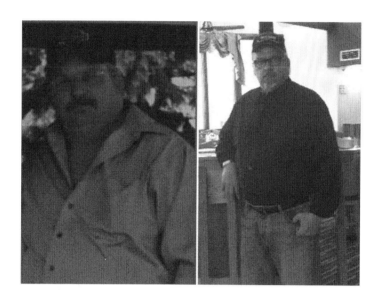

"Sergio's program allows you to find what foods work best for you. I found out which foods I could eat more often, and which to eat on occasion. I love the way I feel and it's not hard to maintain."

—— *Myron B. Lost 141 lbs.*

FOOD SCIENCE & FAT LOSS MYTHS

There is a lot of confusing and conflicting information out there about food, nutrition, and fat loss, even from the so-called experts. So, before we get into the 6 steps to mastering your insulin and jumpstarting your fat loss journey, I want to just share some nutrition science that will help clear some common myths plus help you develop the right mindset to avoid falling for the common diet marketing traps that could lead you back on the path towards frustration and unexplained weight gain.

Ninety-nine percent of the time you are being marketed some weight loss miracle product or system, the company or author is extracting a portion of research without giving you the whole story. That's because absolute and extreme positions are what sells; not science that in the end tells you, "it depends", or that this will work for most people, but not all.

So many of today's nutrition myths have come from these marketing ploys, which come from incomplete research, or they come from folklore. I want you to also understand that many research studies are done on mice or other animals, but have not shown the same impact on humans, or for ethical reasons, the study cannot be performed on humans. Other studies show great short-term results, but over time, the benefits diminish, sometimes even being more harmful in the long run; or often there are no long-term studies. I state this so that you are cautious of programs that claim one quick and simple answer.

Say 'Good-bye' To Belly Fat

Common Myths

- *Counting calories is the most important factor in fat loss*

While maintaining a calorie deficit is critical for weight loss, there are many more factors that impact weight loss and especially fat loss, so you cannot count on calories alone. It's not just calories in versus calorie out because not all calories are created equal. It's pretty obvious that 300 calories from a donut is not the same as 300 calories from a grilled chicken breast and side of broccoli. To start, the thermic effect of foods alone crushes that 'calorie in vs. calorie our' theory. Protein requires about 30 percent of its calories as energy required to simply break it down and digest it, while carbs require about 10 percent, and fats about 3 percent.

Then there's the insulin spike from the donut and its effects including increased fat storage, whereas the protein from the chicken, and carbs and fiber from the broccoli increase metabolism and fat loss. So, while it's important to be in a calorie deficit, there are other critical factors we need to pay attention to in order to be successful losing weight, and especially when its concerning losing belly fat.

- *Large caloric restrictions (Dieting) is the key to weight loss*

Have you or someone you know, gone on a diet and had some success in the first few weeks or months by losing ten or even twenty pounds, only to start feeling fatigued, experience strong cravings, and plateau with

Say 'Good-bye' To Belly Fat

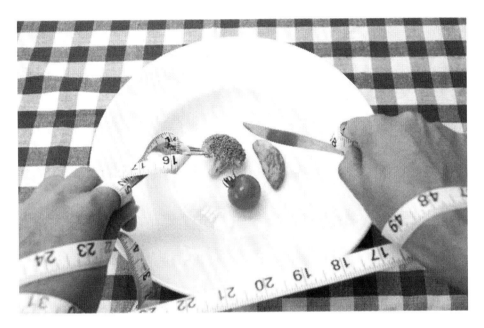

weight loss after just several more weeks or months? There's a reason that over **95 percent of people that go on a diet gain all their weight back plus additional pounds within several months to a year of starting their diet.**

Calories are energy for your body, and if you have too few calories, you will throw your metabolism and hormones out of balance. While it's important to be in a calorie deficit to lose weight, over-restricting your calories and consuming too few calories over time hinders fat loss by slowing your metabolism, throwing hormones out of balance, and causing you to lose muscle density which further slows your metabolism. Long-term calorie restriction (aka dieting) does double damage to your weight loss or fat loss journey by also increasing your risk for high blood pressure and thyroid dysfunction.

Say 'Good-bye' To Belly Fat

- *Carbs are bad for you*

Carbs are NOT bad for you. They are actually essential for good long-term health. The key is to eat primarily whole food complex carbs from vegetables, ancient grains, beans, legumes, and low-glycemic fruit as opposed to processed or simple carbohydrates found in cookies, packaged breads, baked goods, crackers, juices, pasta, and sweets, which spike blood sugars and in turn insulin as well, which then leads to increased fat storage and a whole lot of other issues we'll cover a little later in this book.

The other key is to eat them in the right proportion to the other macros, which depends on your genetics, gut health, current health status, and your weight loss or fat loss goal. But know that complex whole food carbs provide your body and brain with energy, as well as fiber for your digestive system. There are many societies or cultures that consume over 70 percent carbs and have little to no obesity, diabetes, or heart disease.

Cutting out carbs to very low portions like in the Atkins diet (high protein, low carb) or Keto (high fat, low protein, and very low carb) can have short-term benefits, especially when coming from a standard American diet, but so will simply switching out processed simple carbs to natural whole food complex carbs. Both Atkins and Keto have also been shown to have pretty dangerous side effects over time. In many studies, participants on the Atkins Diet ended up gaining all their weight back within 12 months, and we now know that high protein, low carb causes a great deal of inflammation and increases the risk for several chronic diseases including heart disease and certain cancers.

Say 'Good-bye' To Belly Fat

Excess protein also leads to insulin spikes, as well as liver and kidney issues. As for Keto (very high fat, low protein, and very low carb), there have yet to be any long-term research studies beyond 10 years. We are seeing many issues like gut health, cancer, and kidney disease in long-term keto participants. We also know that for a certain percentage of the population that cannot produce enough ketones, this can be an extremely dangerous diet plan. I have two friends that ended up in the hospital within weeks of starting the ketogenic diet. For someone with extreme obesity or diabetes, it may be an effective short-term solution, but it's not the only solution, and it must be done under the guidance of a medical professional. Not indulging on bacon and cheese all day.

- *Fat makes you fat*

This is probably one of the most common nutrition myths that somehow still survives even amongst the plethora of evidence and research against it. Fat does NOT make you fat. Continuous high insulin levels and a caloric surplus make you fat. I think it's still believed by so many people because the American Heart Association (AHA) continues to promote a low-fat diet approach to weight loss and heart health, even though the evidence proves otherwise. In fact, low-fat diets often increase insulin due to removing the fat that would have slowed the absorption and in turn reduced the release of insulin. Then, with the food companies jumping on the AHA bandwagon since the 1980's and making tons of low-fat processed foods loaded with refined carbohydrates, came the obesity, diabetes, and heart disease epidemics.

Say 'Good-bye' To Belly Fat

This version of the low-fat diet is the number one reason obesity, diabetes, and heart disease has spiked somuch over the past 40 years. Please stop buying low-fat yogurt with 18 grams of sugar and a little logo from the AHA that states this food is "heart-healthy". It's NOT.

- *Diet soda is better for you and helps with weight loss*

FALSE! Research shows that even though there is technically zero sugar in diet beverages, blood sugar levels still rise causing insulin to be released. This is due to the negative impact that artificial sweeteners, especially aspartame (Sweet & Low and NutraSweet) and sucralose (Splenda) have on our gut bacteria[1]. Additionally, studies show that we tend to eat more calories (around 20 to 30 percent more) when drinking diet beverages or eating foods with artificial sweeteners, as opposed to naturally sweetened or regular sugar foods and beverages[2]. This is due to our brain's response to the sweetness and an excess release of insulin compared to the minimal sugar spike leading to hypoglycemia (low blood sugars) and stronger food cravings. This effect is even more so for people that are obese, and for women.

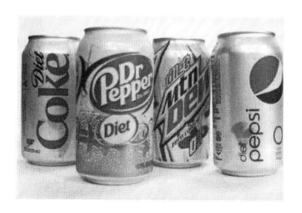

Say 'Good-bye' To Belly Fat

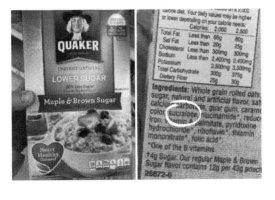

Stevia and monk fruit are two artificial sweeteners with mixed research results. For now, they seem to be the safest, but should only be used occasionally and in moderation. Skip the Diet Coke, Diet Mountain Dew, Gatorade Zero, Powerade Zero, Bang, Celsius, Sugar-Free Red Bull, or other diet beverages. Ideally look for options sweetened with Stevia, or better yet, drink more water and club soda. Additionally, skip foods with aspartame or sucralose like yogurt, instant oatmeal, craisins, canned fruit, ketchup, many cereals.

MASTERING YOUR INSULIN

Now that we've cleared some of the common nutrition myths, let's get to the heart of the matter— managing and mastering your insulin. Following are the 6 steps (or keys) to managing and mastering your insulin to reduce belly fat, kickstart your weight loss, and to help keep it off for good. I've used these over and over with myself and thousands of clients, and it's truly the simplest, healthiest, and most effective long-term weight loss strategy you will find. And you can start putting these steps into practice immediately.

Step 1

MINDFUL EATING

Say 'Good-bye' To Belly Fat

Step 1: MINDFUL EATING

I remember being in my 20's gathering with my friends to watch Michael Jordan and the Chicago Bulls playoff games while enjoying a cold beer and ordering up some deep dish Chicago-style pizza. My mouth watered just thinking of biting into that delicious mound of cheese, sauce, meat, and crust.

When it finally arrived, I would put two slices on my plate, take my first bite and wow- what an explosion of flavor! It was truly a slice of heaven. The second and third bites were pretty amazing too. Then, the next thing I noticed was that I was reloading my plate again with a third and sometimes 4th slice. And somehow, I would finish eating all three or four slices in a matter of just a few minutes without really noticing. Watching the game, talking with my friends, and a few sips of beer, somehow distracted me from fully enjoying one of my all time favorite foods, pizza!

What I would notice is how I wished I could eat one more slice because I wanted to have the same experience from that first bite again, but by that point, I was feeling too stuffed and uncomfortable to have even one more bite. It all went down so fast that I simply couldn't recall if I truly enjoyed the rest of the pizza after the first few bites.

Say 'Good-bye' To Belly Fat

Does any of this sound familiar to you in any way? Mine was pretty extreme, but have you ever plowed through a meal without truly remembering it? That is an example of Unconscious or Mindless eating, which not only leads to overeating, and obviously weight gain, but also has been shown to increase insulin production, and therefore is a double dagger causing additional fat storage and weight gain[3].

Here's another question— *'How often do you eat your food while in a hurry, stressed, or while working?'* If you answered, 'a lot' or 'most meals' or 'all the time', you are not alone; you are actually in the majority. This is really common today, especially in the western world. The problem is that when you are in a hurry, stressed, or working, your body's sympathetic nervous system (fight or flight response) is activated, which in turn shuts down your digestive system and produces cortisol.

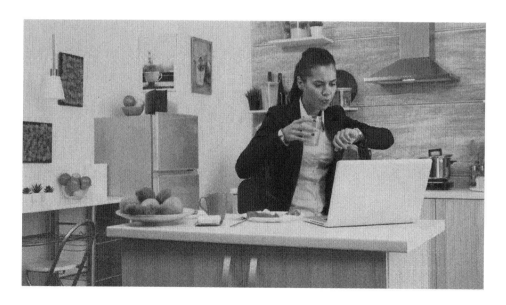

Say 'Good-bye' To Belly Fat

The cortisol that is released into your bloodstream causes glucose (stored sugars) to be released from your muscles to prepare for fight or flight and blocks leptin, the hormone that signals your body when you are full. Well, since you don't ever really go into battle with a jungle beast or have to run for your life, your body releases insulin to bring your blood sugars down again leading to additional fat storage, all while you end up stuffing yourself without noticing until it's too late. It's the perfect recipe for gaining additional weight and belly fat.

There's also the undigested food that ends up passing through without being broken down, so you don't absorb many nutrients, while some of the food simply gets stuck in your digestive tract and begins to putrefy or rot causing gut inflammation that can further lead to additional weight gain as well as serious health issues like IBS, leaky gut, diverticulitis, ulcers, and other conditions.[4]

Have you ever noticed how much more you can eat when you're stressed? How about how easily you can put down an entire bowl of nuts, a bag of chips, and a hot dog or burger while watching a sporting event, not to mention a few beers or cocktails, and not even realize you're full?

Now that you see how eating mindlessly can be preventing you from losing weight and even causing weight gain, let's get into how you can begin to eat mindfully to help *master your insulin* and start losing weight easier and more naturally.

Say 'Good-bye' To Belly Fat

Mindful Eating, Part 1 – Before the meal

Nothing creates pleasure or distracts us from stress like sugar, although it's very temporary. Sugar also comes with many negative consequences, especially when it's in the processed forms of sugar and when consumed frequently. Have you ever noticed what you crave when you're stressed? Usually something sweet like ice cream, cookies, chocolate, or other high-carb (high glucose) foods like bread, chips, or pasta. They take away the stress or pain- for the moment. This is one example of a trigger that we interpret as hunger, but often is not actual hunger, so the first step in practicing mindful eating is to start noticing your triggers, and identifying if you are actually hungry? Especially if you ate a meal or snack less than 3 hours prior, it's most likely not really hunger. Creating a pause between trigger and response is the key to awareness and mindful eating. Get in the habit of doing these 3 steps (responses to hunger triggers) when you first get the signal for a food craving or that you might be hungry.

1. *Take 5 slow deep breaths when you first get a signal that you may be hungry.*

2. *Then drink a glass of water or some tea.*

3. Lastly, set a timer on your phone for 10 minutes and take a walk outside, a stretch break, listen to music, or answer emails- anything that comforts you or distracts you from actually eating. Check in after the ten minutes and notice if are you still feeling hungry or was the trigger connected to something else?

Say 'Good-bye' To Belly Fat

Next, when you are ready to eat, take another five slow deep breaths and ask your body what is it asking for-- what does it truly want to eat. From a reactive or unconscious state, we make habitual choices that are often connected to avoiding pain and seeking pleasure, as I just mentioned, which sugar provides a drip of dopamine to give us that brief experience, so we often make unhealthy choices. From a mindful state, we naturally choose foods that nourish us because survival and wellbeing are our true nature.

Lastly, once you are ready and sitting down to eat, take another five slow deep breaths and spend one to two minutes in gratitude and or prayer for your meal. This will not only prep your body to absorb nutrients and digest better, but also slow you down to be more mindful of when to stop eating.

Mindful Eating, Part 2 – During the meal

As you begin to eat your meal (or snack), spend at least the first two minutes of your meal in full awareness- noticing the colors and textures (sight), the aromas (smell), plus paying attention to all the flavors (taste) and textures (touch) with each bite? Chew slowly and completely (shoot for 30 chews per mouthful) enjoying your food and even noticing how your body feels as you swallow your food and it enters your body. This is great to practice with your kids- you might get a few strange looks, but also a few laughs. How would this experience be different than your current eating habits? Mindful eating also increases insulin sensitivity, which is critical for fat loss.

Say 'Good-bye' To Belly Fat

I can tell you that if you practice this form of mindful eating while eating a giant bowl of pasta and garlic rolls, or a couple of slices of stuffed pizza, or an order of nachos, you will eat less and be able to stop when you are satiated versus stuffed. This habit or skill of 'MINDFUL EATING' not only makes losing belly fat and weight easier, but it makes it easier and more natural to make healthier food choices. It will also change your health and life forever– all by simply being mindful and in-the-moment around choosing and eating your meals.

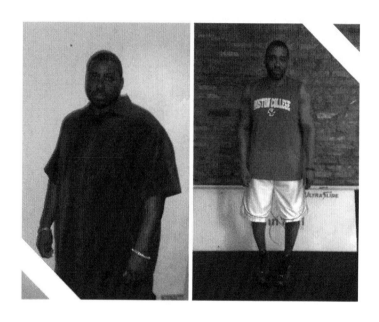

Sergio taught me to pay attention to not only what I was eating, but how I was eating. He also got me to try yoga and now it's a regular part of my routine and lifestyle. This has helped me play basketball better and pain-free

Mike R. Lost 137 lbs.

Say 'Good-bye' To Belly Fat

Karmichael 'Mike' pictured above became a client of mine because I caught him eating unconsciously one day. I don't want to embarrass him, so I won't get into the details about that day, but his willingness to work on these six steps, including "Mindful Eating" truly transformed his life. He not only lost close to 140 pounds, he's kept it off for over 13 years, and he's never going back... because he lives by these principles and steps to mastering his insulin.

These changes have led Mike to practicing Yoga regularly, exercising in ways he enjoys, and playing basketball faster and more athletic without all the major aches and pains from when he weighed close to 400 pounds. This is optimizing your quality of life and why health is so important.

Mindful Eating, Part 3 – After the meal

Mindful Eating doesn't stop when you've finished eating your meal or snack. A key component of "Mindful Eating" is staying mindful and aware of how food affects you AFTER the meal. Food is designed to nourish you — give you energy, strength, improve your cognition, and boost your immune system. Do you feel these benefits from your food, or is it more like the opposite of these and you need an energy drink after your meal? Do you feel fatigued, get brain fog, and feel bloated after your meal? These are often a sign that you are spiking insulin.

So much of today's foods, especially packaged and processed foods, as well as high sodium foods from restaurants, deplete your energy and even your nourishment. These foods are actually killing you by not only

Say 'Good-bye' To Belly Fat

damaging and destroying your cells, including your immune system's T-cells, but also by spiking insulin, which again is connected to all chronic diseases. It's no big mystery why Americans are getting sicker younger and taking prescription medications earlier in life than ever before.

Paying attention to how your body feels for a couple of hours after a meal can give you important information on whether a particular food is nourishing you and providing you with energy or if it's causing inflammation, destroying your health, and possibly spiking insulin. Sometimes even healthy foods like broccoli, cauliflower, or almonds, may not be good specifically for you. We all have a unique microbiome, genetics, and current health state that dictate our response to foods, which can cause us to not break down and digest certain foods properly and therefore have reactions like bloating, diarrhea, mental fogginess, or fatigue from specific foods.

Because we have become used to feeling bloated and or fatigued after meals, it takes a little practice to begin to truly notice how foods affect you. Ideally, a Food Sensitivity Test and a continuous glucose monitor (CGM) are two tools that give you accurate information on your body's response to certain foods. These are a bit pricey and not easily accessible for everyone, so I want to teach you the steps to do this on your own.

To practice this habit, pay attention to how you are feeling immediately after the meal, and for the next two to three hours by asking yourself these five questions (do this daily for at least three weeks and track it using the Daily Mindful Eating Tracker in the back of this book):

POST-MEAL QUESTIONS FOR MINDFUL EATING

- 1. **Do I have more energy and mental clarity or less energy and feel mentally foggy?**

    2. **Does my stomach feel bloated?**

    3. **Do I feel satiated for at least 3 to 4 hours, or do I get cravings soon after, or feel hungry again less than 3 hours after a meal?**

    4. **Does my mood change and become more irritable?**

    5. **Does my skin itch or turn red in spots?**

These five questions will help you identify the foods that work best for YOU. If you get a negative response to a meal, you may need to separate the different food items in your meal and try to identify which of the foods is causing the issue. Common foods that can cause reactions are processed meats, dairy, refined sugar, corn, wheat, and caffeine.

Practicing Mindful Eating is the first step in helping you master your insulin and reducing belly fat in a way that supports not only long-term weight loss but also living a healthy lifestyle.

Say 'Good-bye' To Belly Fat

ACTION PLAN SUMMARY for MINDFUL EATING:

When you first begin to think about eating or something triggers a desire for food, take 5 deep breaths and be fully present in your body- what is it really asking for? If you are aware that you are craving something unhealthy and a part of you is telling you not to have it, then have a glass of water, take a few more deep breaths, and set your timer for 10 minutes. Then recheck with your body.

When you sit down to eat your food, take 60 to 90 seconds and do more slow deep breathing while you pray over your food, or simply spend time in gratitude over your food before eating.

Eat super slow and mindfully, especially for the first few minutes. Be fully present and chew completely (30 times with each mouthful) while noticing taste, textures, smells, colors, sounds, and even your body's sensations as food enters your body. Put the food or fork down between bites. Enjoy the meal by being fully present and stop eating when you are feeling satiated and no longer hungry.

Pay attention for the next several hours after your meal and notice if your energy and mental clarity go up or down; if your mood gets any better or worse; if you feel bloating; if your skin has any reactions; and if you get cravings or feel hungry again in less than three hours. Ideally, you will want to journal what you ate and how your body and mind responded to every meal for a few weeks to help you really understand what foods serve you best, and which you should minimize or avoid altogether. Use the tracker at the end of the book to help you.

Say 'Good-bye' To Belly Fat

The challenging part of Mindful Eating is that we've become so accustomed to feeling bloated, mentally foggy, fatigued, etc... that's it's become our norm. I promise you that it's not the normal, nor is it healthy. I remember when I first began coaching truck drivers and they started implementing some of the six steps in this book, and how amazed they were at how different and how much better they felt. They didn't even know it was possible. Many drivers and other clients even gave up caffeine because they started having so much more energy from the food they were eating. Imagine that- your food giving you energy.

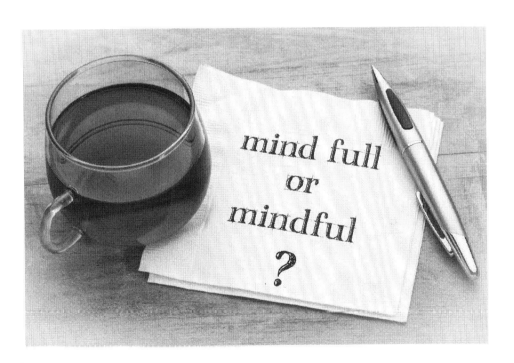

Step 2

Get Gut Healthy

Step 2. GET GUT HEALTHY

Do you ever eat a specific food, and your belly just seems to get bloated by several inches in what seems to be an instant? Or do certain foods make you *RUN* to the bathroom, sometimes in a state of panic? Do you have certain foods that cause you to have skin reactions, or do you struggle with an auto-immune disease? These are all signs that your gut health is compromised and there's a high probability that it's affecting your ability to lose fat, as well as likely causing you to store extra fat, among other other health concerns, including a higher risk of many chronic diseases and emotional health issues.

The microbiome (gut bacteria) in your digestive system is the foundation of your metabolism and the first point in your body that dictates what your body will do with the calories you just consumed. Poor gut health leads to inflammation, and inflammation leads to poor gut health. It's a negative cycle that needs to be corrected since poor gut health not only prevents fat loss, but it can also cause weight gain[5]. Poor gut health is also connected to an increased risk of developing diabetes and heart disease[6] since it negatively impacts our ability to manage insulin by reducing butyrate[7]. Furthermore, it can cause you to feel hungry even when you are not by disrupting the signals from leptin, ghrelin, and other peptides that signal your body when you're full. Without that signal you often end up eating beyond your hunger point without noticing and is just one of the many reasons that poor gut health is connected to obesity[8].

Say 'Good-bye' To Belly Fat

To top it off, poor gut health also leads to disrupted sleep as well as reduced cognition and mood. Yes- an unhealthy gut can contribute to the inability to focus, to feeling cranky, and even depressed.

I hope you now see the importance of having good gut health, not only for losing belly fat and weight, but also for all the health implications connected to your gut. And if that's still not enough to motivate you, did you know that between 70 and 80 percent of your immune system is in your gut. Yes, poor gut health is connected to a compromised immune system? With what we've been seeing with the pandemic in 2020 and 2021, I believe it's more essential today than ever to have a strong and healthy immune system. Let's look at several simple steps to improving your gut health.

Variety is the Spice of Life

One way to begin improving your gut bacteria is to make sure you are consuming a variety of foods. Avoid getting caught up in the routine of eating mostly the same foods every day. I've seen pro athletes and bodybuilders get stuck on eating the same foods every day for months and even years. While they look great due to their extreme fitness regimen, many have developed serious gut health issues, and end up gaining a bunch of weight when their careers end because the exercise regimen isn't there to overcome the gut issues. Same with many people that go on diets.

The key here is to focus on getting a wide variety of whole foods, including a variety of vegetables, fruits, nuts, seeds, whole or ancient grains, beans, lentils, and a little bit of natural, hormone-free dairy and wild meats. Traditionally raised and processed dairy and meats, especially red meat, can cause gut bacteria imbalances and issues. Otherwise, think of eating the rainbow, which you've probably heard that phrase once or twice.

Poly-Pheno-menal

Make sure to eat lots of plant-based foods and herbs like artichoke, parsley, strawberries, asparagus, apples, broccoli, carrots, berries, grapefruit, black beans, tofu, flaxseeds, almonds, walnuts, cinnamon, cumin, and many others that are rich in polyphenols to help the colon. I recommend lightly cooked vegetables, especially if you have gut issues, since they are often easier on the gut. If you currently have a diagnosed gut issue like IBS, or experience regular gut discomfort, make sure to speak with your medical doctor about which vegetables are acceptable and which are not specifically for you.

Not-So-Sweet

Sugar may taste sweet, but it's not so sweet or kind to your body, your brain, and your gut when you consume more than your body needs. Excess sugar is a major disruptor to your gut health by feeding your 'unhealthy' or 'bad' bacteria causing inflammation and increased cravings for more sugar[9]. Have you ever noticed after having a cookie, how much stronger the craving is for the 2nd and 3rd cookies? It's an uphill battle if you want to stop eating more cookies. Here's an interesting and crazy fact — one hundred years ago, Americans consumed an average of 4 pounds of sugar per year. Today, the average American consumes... (guess)

Say 'Good-bye' To Belly Fat

...over 150 pounds of sugar each year! 150 lbs. of SUGAR!!

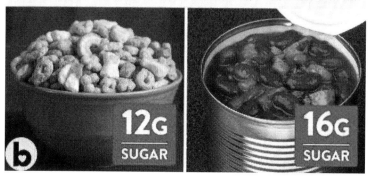

How crazy is that? One reason for the excess in sugar consumption is that we've switched from eating mostly home-cooked all natural whole foods to mostly buying and eating packaged and processed foods. And with an estimated 74 percent of foods containing added sugars[10], it's easy to see how we've gone into a major sugar overdose. We think added sugars are only in desserts like cakes, cookies, and candy, but if you start reading food labels, you'll find added sugars in all kinds of foods like breads, pasta, canned beans, tomato sauces, ketchup, salad dressings, instant oatmeal, yogurt, and so many others.

Many of these are even promoted as 'healthy' foods, but they're far from it[11]. The second reason we are now consuming 40X more sugar than we were 100 years ago is that we have also become a snacking society. We want to snack all day—we've even been told that it's best to eat six small meals versus the traditional three square meals, which was based on incomplete science. While eating smaller, more frequent meals does speed up your metabolism a bit, it's minimal and only lasts a few months. After five to six months, there is no benefit, and in fact, you're more likely to have caused inflammation and imbalance to your gut bacteria. It's more beneficial for our gut bacteria to eat three square meals, or two meals and a snack, so there is longer breaks between meals. But when you do really want a snack, it's best to snack on something natural like a handful of nuts and seeds, or a piece of low-glycemic fruit like an apple, or a cup of berries with a little Greek yogurt or cottage cheese. Stay away from packaged snacks, even the "100- calorie" snacks which are mostly loaded with sugar.

Lastly, avoid artificial sweeteners, which we discussed above in the Nutrition Myths section. These do even more damage to your gut health, as well as damage insulin receptors and cause insulin to spike.

Pre-biotics

Unlike probiotics, which are living micro-organisms found in fermented foods that do wonders for our digestive system and our immune system, prebiotics are compounds in our foods that we cannot digest but are a good source of food for our microbiome, our probiotics. This 'good' bacteria in your gut cannot survive without its own food source, which comes in the form of pre-biotics from certain foods like Jerusalem artichoke, apples, asparagus, bananas, cabbage, dandelion, garlic, mushroom, oats, and others.

Say 'Good-bye' To Belly Fat

Focused Fiber

We've all been told to 'eat your fiber', except for Keto folks- they somehow don't believe much in fiber. I'll save that for another discussion, so for now, let me explain what fiber even is since I get asked often. Fiber is a specific type of carbohydrate within certain foods that our bodies cannot easily digest, so it passes through the digestive tract quickly without raising blood sugar levels. More specifically, there are two types of fiber, soluble and insoluble fiber that together make what we call dietary fiber (DT).

Soluble fiber forms a gel-like substance that passes through into the colon providing food for the gut bacteria in the large intestine and has been shown to reduce the risk of colon cancer[12] among many other health benefits like blocking fat absorption making it a strong ally in helping you lose weight. Insoluble fiber does not dissolve, nor can we absorb or digest it, so it acts more like a sweeper of the digestive tract cleaning the intestine walls and helping you to stay regular.

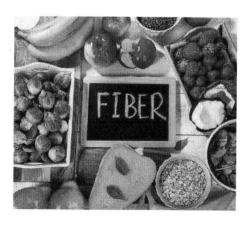

Say 'Good-bye' To Belly Fat

Dietary fiber is your friend. It increases insulin sensitivity and keeps you feeling full longer, both of which will help you tremendously on your weight loss journey. It also improves gut health, immune health, heart health (lowers cholesterol and increases insulin sensitivity), and cognitive function[13].

Ideally, you want to shoot for 30 to 40 grams of fiber per day, but first make sure you track your average amount of daily fiber, and increase by no more than 5 grams of fiber daily every five to seven days. When you consider the Standard American Diet (SAD), which really is sad, and sometimes called the 'Western' Diet, this dietary lifestyle is filled with processed carbs, lots of processed protein, hormone-filled dairy, and very little fiber. Most Americans get an average of 10 to 15 grams of fiber per day, which is less than half of what is recommended. And we wonder why obesity and heart disease are increasing in epidemic proportions in our country and the 'western' world.

Aside from specific foods, which I'll cover in the next step/chapter (Manage Your Macros), you can get fiber supplements to add to smoothies, yogurt, or even a cookie or pancake batter to make them healthier and reduce or prevent insulin spikes

PRO-biotics

The Pros that really get your gut healthy are the micro-organisms that come from fermented foods and transfer into your intestines and provide a myriad of health benefits including increasing your metabolism, which of course is connected to weight loss. Some of the most probiotic-friendly foods are kimchi, organic Greek yogurt, tempeh, miso, kombucha tea, and pickles. You can also take a high-quality probiotic every other day to help improve your gut health.

Get Your Z's

Sleep is one of the most studied areas within the health and wellness space over the past 30 years. Poor sleep is not only linked to poor gut health, but also weight gain, diabetes, heart disease, and dementia. Adults should be getting at least 7 hours of sleep. Not getting enough sleep disrupts our microbiome, which in turn further disrupts our sleep. To get better sleep, practice proper sleep hygiene like sleeping and waking at or around the same time every day; limiting caffeine at least six to ten hours before bedtime; avoiding blue light after sundown; sleeping in complete darkness; and keeping room temperature cool during sleep. I'll discuss sleep hygiene in more detail in a later section since it is one of the keys to managing insulin.

ACTION PLAN SUMMARY to GET YOUR GUT HEALTHY:

Eat a variety of foods— don't get caught in the pattern of eating mostly the same foods on most days. Also eat mostly vegetables, nuts, seeds, lentils, beans, whole and ancient grains, some fruits, and a little organic dairy and wild-caught fish and meats

Say 'Good-bye' To Belly Fat

Get lots of high polyphenol foods like artichoke, parsley, strawberries, asparagus, apples, broccoli, carrots, berries, grapefruit, black beans, tofu, flaxseeds, almonds, walnuts, cinnamon, cumin, and many others

Eat mostly natural whole foods and minimize or avoid packaged foods with added sugars. Snack on natural foods like nuts and seeds or low-glycemic fruit. For packaged foods, try foods like Primal Kitchen brand which do not add sugars.

Get prebiotic foods like Jerusalem artichoke, apples, asparagus, bananas, cabbage, dandelion, garlic, mushroom, oats, and others.

Eat foods rich in fiber like beans, lentils, avocados, berries, whole grains, apples, broccoli, sweet potato, nuts... ARE YOU STARTING TO SEE A PATTERN OF HEALTHY FOODS? Shoot for 30 to 40 grams of fiber daily, but increase gradually (no more than 5 grams increase every three to five days).

Eat Probiotic-rich foods like kimchi, organic Greek yogurt, tempeh, miso, kombucha tea, and pickles.

Get a minimum of 7 hours of sleep and follow proper sleep hygiene.

Improving your gut health is the second step or key to mastering your insulin. By putting these micro-habits into practice that improve your microbiome, you will be closer to mastering your insulin, plus experience less bloating, more mental and physical energy, better sleep, and accelerated weight loss.

Step 3

Manage Your Macros

Step 3: MANAGE YOUR MACROS

'How much protein should I have?' 'Should I eat carbs?' How many grams of fat are in this?' These are just a few of the hundreds of questions you may have asked yourself at one point or another- or may still be asking yourself today about macros. I want to emphasize two key points here.

First, there is no macro ratio that works best for everyone. We are all unique with different microbiome, genetics, and current health state, so it's a process to discover ratios that are are ideal for you that will provide you with energy and help with fat loss and weight loss.

Second, more important than your macro ratios, is the quality of your macros. Protein from a chicken breast that comes from a traditional factory-farmed chicken that you find in most restaurants, just about every fast-food restaurant, and even most grocery stores, is not the same as the protein from chicken that is naturally raised and free from hormones and antibiotics. Same as carbs from lentils and wild rice are not the same as carbs from white bread or a cookie. And fat from an avocado is not the same fat as fat from fast food ground beef. The quality of your macros is paramount to your body and system, including your insulin.

When it comes to macros, you most likely think about protein, carbs, fat, and possibly fiber, but we're also going to add in water and alcohol, which Shawn Stevenson in his book "Eat Smarter" does a great job of showing

Say 'Good-bye' To Belly Fat

how these macro-nutrients play such a big role in our overall health. He uses the analogy of these six as the players on a basketball team with fiber being the utility 6th man. Adding to his analogy of a basketball team, I will add that the top goal for this team is to manage insulin by keeping it within a healthy range as often and for as long as possible. And all six players (the entire team) have to do their part to make this goal happen.

As I mentioned earlier, macros play a critical role in managing your blood glucose, and therefore can wreak havoc on your insulin if they're not managed properly. But your insulin response is also based on your unique genetics, body composition, gut health, and metabolism, so while a food may be labeled as 'low-glycemic' (meaning it doesn't spike blood glucose too much), or you may be enjoying a 'low-carb' meal, you may have a significant sugar and insulin response to that food, as it did for several participants in a research study[14]. On the contrary, you may want to treat yourself to a bowl of pasta or a cookie thinking you shouldn't because it will spike blood glucose and insulin, but in fact, you're blessed with the right genes and metabolism, that they don't spike insulin much at all. In the mentioned study, researchers compared the glucose response to a banana and compared it to the glucose response of a cookie. While most participants in the study had the expected response of low sugar spikes to the banana and high sugar spikes to the cookie, there were several participants that had the opposite response. This study has been duplicated with a variety of foods showing more variation in in responses to foods.

Say 'Good-bye' To Belly Fat

This is why practicing 'Mindful Eating' will help you tremendously in noticing your insulin response to foods. An energy crash, food coma, or strong food cravings usually equates to a high insulin spike. You may choose to wear a continuous glucose monitor to know for sure, but it's not practical for everyone, although they are now available over the counter, which is a great because you used to need a prescription in order to get one. Now let's take a look at each of the macros and learn how we can better understand them to help us master insulin and jumpstart weight loss.

PROTEIN

Protein is highly regarded by most but underutilized and misunderstood. In other words, most people know and talk about getting a good amount of protein, but very few people do. Aside from being the building block for muscle tissue, protein also helps with regulating blood glucose, manage insulin, burn fat, and manage your appetite—all of which stimulate fat loss. One more fat loss bonus is that protein has a high thermic effect requiring between around 30 percent of its calories to be burned as fuel simply to break it down and digest it (carbs require about 10 percent and fat requires around 3 percent).

In fact, there have been several studies that show by increasing protein alone, while leaving calories constant, participants experienced significant weight loss and reduction of body-fat[13]. But, before you go out and buy a bunch of steaks, chicken breasts, and protein powders, it's important to note three things.

Say 'Good-bye' To Belly Fat

1. Too much protein can create lots of health issues like constipation, kidney damage, dehydration (the first five to fifteen pounds of weight loss on the Atkins diet is mostly water weight), heart disease, loss of calcium, certain cancers, and even weight gain. Too much protein can also create insulin spikes.

2. Get protein from a variety of sources to get the best benefits including weight loss and keeping your gut healthy. Wild animal protein (much better than farmed), nuts and seeds, eggs, tempeh/tofu, beans, lentils, ancient grains like amaranth and quinoa, Greek yogurt, Grass-fed whey protein isolate, and pea protein powder are some of your best sources.

3. As I stated earlier, **quality matters more than you think**. Read that again please. If you eat animal protein, wild-caught animal protein like venison, bison, fish and wild game are by far your best bet. Beef should be organic plus grass-fed and finished. Chicken, turkey, and pork should be 100 percent naturally raised or wild. Did you know that 80 percent of antibiotics in this country are given to farmed animals, not humans? These antibiotics are passed down to us when we eat these meats, causing damage to our digestive system and gut flora, which we discussed in the last chapter, among other health risks. So, be cautious and avoid or limit protein from fast food, restaurant chains, and even many grocers. Many buy the left-over scrubs then add a bunch of salt to mask their taste. Eatwild.com and U.S. Wellness Meats **are two**

Say 'Good-bye' To Belly Fat

great resources for high quality proteins.

Now that we covered quality, let's discuss ratios. While everyone is individual and there is no one diet or macro ratio that works best for everyone, there is a great deal of research that supports starting out at 25 to 30 percent of your caloric intake. For example, if you eat 2,000 calories per day, 25 to 30 percent will equal 500 to 600 of the calories coming from protein. And since each gram of protein is 4 calories, that will equal 125 to 150g of protein per day. This is a good starting point knowing you can adjust up or down a little to find your sweet spot for energy, digestion, and weight loss. Your level of physical activity will also dictate your demand for protein. Sadly, with the Standard American Diet (SAD), Americans are only getting an average of 10 to 20 percent of their calories from protein, and it's usually very poor quality protein.

Over 46 percent of American adults don't even get the RDA minimum of 10 percent.

CARBS

This is by far the most debated macro-nutrient of the bunch. There are advocates and research supporting both sides of the coin, on whether carbs cause weight gain or not. I will try and keep this as simple as possible because it is more complex than simply asking 'do carbs cause weight gain?' It is absolutely true that carbs alone do not cause weight gain, but it's also not just calories in versus calories out as we've already cleared up. It's elevated insulin levels that inhibit weight loss, and elevated insulin levels over time that cause fat storage and weight gain. Carbs are just one piece of the puzzle but can play a major role in insulin response for most people. But please know that carbs do not impact insulin the same for everyone. There are populations like the Kitavan's, Pima Indians, or Okinawan's that have diets consisting of 70 to 85 percent carbohydrates that don't experience elevated insulin levels, nor do they have obesity, diabetes, or heart disease. Again, quality is a huge factor.

For most people, especially in the western world, eating the wrong type of carbs, above our personal threshold, and or at the wrong time, often leads to elevated insulin levels. And as I mentioned before, elevated insulin levels over time leads to insulin resistance, excess fat storage, weight gain, and other metabolic health issues including high cholesterol, high blood pressure, and pre-diabetes or diabetes. It's more a matter of how the type, amount, and timing of the carbs affect you personally, which is dictated by genetics, your microbiome, and your current health status, including if you're overweight or obese, and for how long.

Without labeling carbs 'good' or 'bad' carbs, I prefer to describe them as simple carbs (think white bread, crackers, cookies, cakes chips, candy, fruit juices, and pasta) and complex carbs like vegetables, leafy greens, whole grains, beans, lentils, and low-glycemic fruits. Simple carbs, which are often refined and processed are far more likely to cause weight gain by causing gut health issues, increased hunger and food cravings, and

Say 'Good-bye' To Belly Fat

often causing insulin to spike[16], whereas complex carbs provide your body and brain with energy, fuel for your cells, help regulate hormones, and often pack along a good amount of fiber, which we saw earlier is critical for gut health, among other health benefits.

So, now that you know complex carbs are the better choice, how do you know how much the right amount for you is? Without a continuous glucose monitor, which is ideal but not practical for most of us, you need to rely on your own awareness and mindfulness to notice how foods are affecting you. That's why "Mindful Eating' is the first step and key to *mastering your insulin*. You will notice that when you go over your threshold for carbs, you will notice energy crashes, hormone dysfunction, hunger cravings, and weight gains. I recommend starting with 40 to 45 percent of your calories coming from complex carbs. With the 2,000 calorie example, that would equal to 200 to 225 grams of carbs per day. if your daily caloric intake is 1,700 calories, then you would consume between 170 and 190 grams of carbs per day. Pay attention to your energy, hunger, food cravings, weight loss or weight gain, and sleep. Increase and decrease your carb intake as needed.

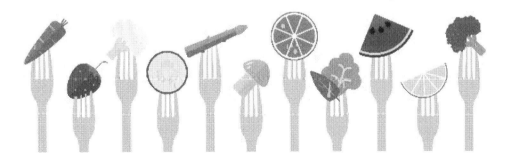

Say 'Good-bye' To Belly Fat

Once per week, allow yourself to indulge a bit and increase your carb intake to 50 to 55 percent of your caloric intake, but still try and get most from complex carbs. An occasional treat like a cookie or cake is fine; the challenge is what happens to your brain as a response— you feel like you need 2 more; and then 3 more; and so on, so be very mindful.

One trick you can do to reduce the strong sugar response and cravings for more when you want to have a sweet treat is to have it with protein or some healthy fats. I often have a handful of walnuts or a ½ a protein shake when I know I want a little chocolate or a slice of key lime pie. My daughter also makes our own home-made pancakes with banana, oats, protein powder, ground flax seed, and an egg, plus drizzles peanut butter on top with the maple syrup to make them a much healthier version that won't spike blood glucose too much.

Lastly, the timing of carbs is very important. Most importantly, do not eat a carb-loaded meal as your first meal of the day. One of the worst things you can do is start your day with high glycemic cereal and milk (which is a carb, and the lower the fat of the milk, the higher the glycemic index), a bagel, or other baked goods and a high sugar coffee drink. For most people, this will increase sugar cravings and hunger throughout the day. Instead, start your day with some low glycemic fruit and protein like cottage cheese, Greek yogurt, or eggs. Bagels, muffins, pancakes, waffles, and other high-carb foods should be saved for special occasions or limited to once or twice per month. Having complex carbs at lunch and even at dinner is totally fine and can even improve sleep.

Say 'Good-bye' To Belly Fat

As far as the relationship to exercise, contrary to most people's belief, it's better to consume carbs post-workout, not pre-workout. Exercising without carbs (either fasting or with a little protein) will cause your body to utilize fat for fuel quicker. And then taking in some carbs (with some protein and fat) post-workout since our insulin sensitivity is at its peak.

FAT

We covered Fat a little bit in our "Myths" section. This is probably the second most debated macro-nutrient, and that is mostly due to the promotion and marketing craze over the Ketogenic diet, and the opposing view and push by the American Heart Association's for a low-fat diet as the best means for not only heart health but also for weight loss, which there is far more evidence supporting the contrary. Cutting out fat from your diet has not been shown to help in weight loss, and has often resulted in weight gain, especially when replacing fat with low-fat processed foods.

It's also important to know that there are various types of fat— saturated fat (which can be broken down into long, medium, and short-chain), monounsaturated fats, and polyunsaturated fats. Each of these types of fats provides different benefits, and it's important to have a balanced variety of each of these in your diet.

While fat does NOT make you fat, there are a few key items about fats that are critical to overall health and healthy fat loss.

Say 'Good-bye' To Belly Fat

Saturated fats are NOT bad fats. The medium-chain and short-chain saturated fatty acids in particular (goat's milk, coconut fat, ghee, butter, certain cheeses) have loads of health benefits including reducing inflammation and reducing visceral fat (the dangerous fat around your organs). This is the belly fat you want to say 'Good-bye' to more than anything, and the main reason I wrote this book.

Foods with high monounsaturated fats (think olives, olive oil, avocadoes, avocado oil, nuts like Brazilian nuts, cashews, macadamia nuts, and pumpkin seeds) have been shown to help lower blood glucose levels and improve insulin sensitivity, which is key to *mastering your insulin*. Monounsaturated fats have also been shown to improve cholesterol and curb cravings.

PUFAs or polyunsaturated fats are found in most nuts, seeds, fish, beef, and some plant-based oils. Omega-3 and omega-6 are the popular and most notable of the polyunsaturated fats. It's important to get a good amount of each with a ratio between 2:1 and 3:1 of omega 6 to omega 3, which helps reduce inflammation and improve cholesterol. The issue here is that most Americans get a ratio of around 17:1 of omega-6 to omega-3 ratio with some folks getting as bad as a 50:1, which increases inflammation and can lead to weight gain and even heart disease. Worse yet, Americans get the vast majority of their omega-6's in the form of highly processed vegetable oils (corn, cottonseed, safflower, soybean) from packaged foods. Due to PUFA's instability, when exposed to high heat, such as cooking with them or the processing of packaged foods, they become highly oxidized and lead to hardening of our arteries more than saturated fat from steak.

○

Omega-3 healthy foods include mackerel, salmon, cod liver, oysters, sardine, anchovies, flaxseed, and chia seeds.

○

Omega-6 healthy foods include walnuts, safflower oil, tofu, hemp seeds, sunflower seeds, avocado oil, almonds, cashews, and natural nut butters like peanut butter, almond butter, and cashew butter.

There are loads of foods with healthy fats essential for good health and mastering insulin like extra virgin olive oil, avocados, fatty fish, nuts, full fat or 2% organic Greek yogurt, eggs, dark chocolate (over 70% cacao), and certain cheeses.

FIBER

We already covered fiber in our "Gut Health" section, but as a quick reminder, shoot for 30 to 40 grams of fiber per day. Do not increase by more than 3 to 5 grams every several days. Too much fiber too fast will cause discomfort, bloating, and emergency sprints to the bathroom. On the bright side, it may encourage you to get some sprints in. Joking aside, increase your fiber gradually, but make sure you are getting enough fiber.

Say 'Good-bye' To Belly Fat

Here are a few foods that are loaded with fiber:

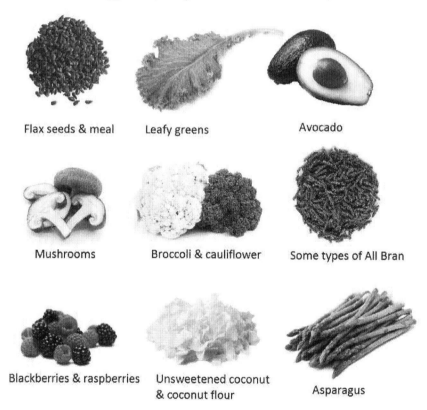

Lentils, Chickpeas, Apples, Kidney Beans, Chia seeds, Pistachios, Pears, Fresh coconut, Sunflower seeds, Oats

Quinoa, Sweet Potato, Split Peas, Artichoke, Blackberries, Mushrooms, Flaxseed, Avocados

Say 'Good-bye' To Belly Fat

WATER

Most people never discuss water as a macro-nutrient, but I promise you, it's a critical macro- nutrient and has many benefits including improving metabolism and digestion, so you want to make sure it's a significant part of your daily intake. While there's no science behind the popular suggestion of 64 ounces, I think it's a good starting point for most people. If you weigh over 175 pounds, I recommend adding 16 to 32 more ounces. Depending on how much you sweat, you may need to add more water, especially if exercising for more than 30 minutes, or performing high-intensity exercise. Lastly, for every 8 ounces of caffeinated beverage, you should add 16 ounces of water. The key is once you feel thirsty, it's too late and you went too long without water.

Some of the major health benefits of water include:

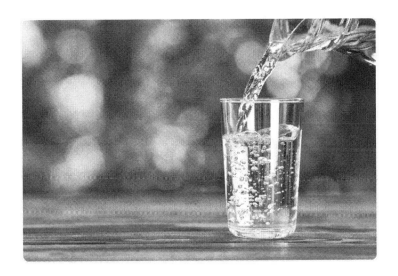

Say 'Good-bye' To Belly Fat

1. Carries nutrients and oxygen to your cells Normalizes blood pressure

2. Helps flush out toxins

3. Aids digestion

4. Help you stay regular Helps produce saliva

5. Protects joints and muscles

6. Helps control appetite

If you struggle drinking plain water, try infusing it with fruits, vegetables, and herbs. Avoid adding flavor drops, especially if they are sweetened with sucralose or aspartame. Here are some of my favorite infused water recipes:

Strawberry, Basil, Lemon

Cucumber & Mint (honeydew – optional)

Grapefruit, Pomegranate, Mint

Blackberries, Orange, Ginger

Watermelon, Kiwi, Lime

Pineapple, Coconut, Lime

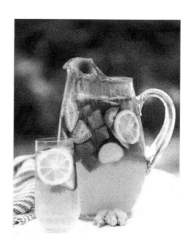

Say 'Good-bye' To Belly Fat

ALCOHOL

Alcohol plays a significant role in energy production, but also comes with major consequences. I am not here to tell you not to have any alcoholic drinks— I enjoy a glass of wine or whiskey every once in a while, myself. But I do want you to understand how it impacts fat loss, as well as overall health when drinking alcohol.

Alcohol is a drug and it's highly addictive, so first and foremost, be mindful and seek help if you feel you are not in control. Research shows that limiting to 1 to 1.5 drinks per day on average, with at least one day of non-drinking per week, can have some health benefits. But because alcohol inhibits all other forms of energy expenditure, it can lead to rapid weight gains, especially around the belly, if drinking more than your threshold, which again is dictated by your genes, microbiome, and current health.

Please note that most alcohol negatively impacts gut health with the exception of 1 to 1.5 glasses of red wine, unless you are sensitive to tannins, which then even red wine might also cause harm to your gut bacteria. If your skin gets a little red and or you feel your body temperature rise a bit when you drink red wine or any alcohol, that particular beverage is causing you additional damage, so I recommend avoiding it, or only for very special occasions if you truly enjoy it. Drinking 2 or more drinks on average per day is linked to obesity as well as other health issues like heart disease, liver disease, and even dementia.

Say 'Good-bye' To Belly Fat

If you've plateaued with your weight loss, especially the last ten to fifteen pounds or you are more than thirty pounds overweight, I highly suggest avoiding alcohol for at least three weeks (or longer if you wish). Ideally, make it part of a complete sugar detox, where you avoid all foods with added sugars. This will help improve your gut health plus allow your liver to reset itself and become more effective, which in turn will help you burn more fat and boost your metabolism.

There are 7g of sugar for every ounce of alcohol, so the sugars can add up quickly. Additionally, most alcoholic beverages can pack on the calories very quickly. For example, most beers are between 150 and 250 calories and 12 to 20 grams of carbs, with light beers being between 90 and 140 calories and between 2.5 (ultra-light) and 9 grams of carbs. A 5 oz. glass of wine carries 120 to 140 calories and around 4 grams of carbs. Hard seltzers come in low-calorie and low-carb options, but again, more than one or two packs on empty calories.

One of the best ways to indulge is to have vodka or tequila with club soda. Adding bitters will accent the flavor, plus increase your sensitivity to insulin, which is a little pre-meal hack if you are out to dinner and want to have a drink before the food arrives.

Say 'Good-bye' To Belly Fat

ACTION PLAN SUMMARY to MANAGE YOUR MACROS

Now that you have a good sense of all the macros and the important roles they play, you might be wondering what's the best ratios you should be eating to lose weight and more importantly, belly fat? Well, of course, that depends— on your gut health, genetics, metabolism, and current health condition.

More important than measuring macro ratios is getting clean high-quality protein, complex carbs, a variety of healthy fats, 30 to 40 grams of fiber, plenty of water, and minimize alcohol. Measuring and tracking your ratios does have some great benefits and doesn't have to be done forever. The key is to get an understanding of what specific foods, calories, and macro ratios work best specifically for you. With that said, if it seems too stressful and overwhelming, then by all means, don't worry about it. I've had many clients lose belly fat and weight without tracking their macros or even counting calories. How? By eating Mindful and sticking to predominantly whole, real, natural foods. Here are a few key takeaways regarding macros and macro ratios...

If the majority of your calories come from whole, real, unprocessed foods, your gut health, metabolism, energy, and sleep will all improve— all things that help with weight loss, so the macro ratios will not be as critical, especially if you are less than 25 pounds overweight.

Say 'Good-bye' To Belly Fat

If you'd like to track macros to see what ratios work best for you, a good starting point for most people is 30% protein, 45% carbs (as long as these are complex natural whole food carbs), and 25% fat. Be mindful and pay attention to energy, weight gain or loss, food cravings, sleep, etc… Make adjustments as necessary starting with adjusting fat and carbs but leaving protein between 25 and 30 percent.

If you are more than 25 pounds overweight, you can still try the above ratios (30-45-25), with whole foods and stay in a caloric deficit, but if you don't experience weight loss or reduction in belly fat after two or three weeks, try decreasing your carbs to 30 percent and increasing your fat to 40 percent (remember healthy fats: fish, nuts, avocados, olives and olive oil, etc…), while keeping your protein the same at 30 percent. This has been a successful model for many, but it always depends on your metabolic type as well as gut health, genetics, and current health condition. If this causes an energy dip, discomfort, or weight gain for longer than a few days, you may be a slow oxidizer and do better with more carbs. If that is the case, reduce your protein to 20 to 25 percent, increase your carbs to 55%, and 20 to 25 percent fat. This part is always an exploration since we are all unique. The critical message here is to prioritize Mindful Eating, Gut Health, and real whole natural foods.

Step 4

FASTING

Step 4: FASTING

Fasting has been practiced since the beginning of time, although not always by choice. Hunters and gatherers would go days without eating because they couldn't find food. Throughout history, there have also been times of famine and very little food. Aside from these, almost all religions practice some form of fasting as a spiritual practice.

Dozens of studies have shown that fasting is effective for weight loss[17], although not much different than calorie restriction. The real difference is that fasting improves insulin sensitivity and metabolism, which results in far better long-term fat loss and weight loss benefits, in addition to all the other health benefits we mentioned that are connected to regulating insulin.

Additionally, there are studies that fasting helps with longevity due to stimulating cellular autophagy, as well as stem cell and human growth hormone production. It's also been shown to reduce symptoms of chemotherapy treatment in many cancer patients

The three most popular forms of intermittent fasting are Alternate-Day Fasting, 5:2 Fasting, and Time-Restricted.

Say 'Good-bye' To Belly Fat

1. **Alternate Day Fasting** consists of abstaining from eating any calories every other day. You simply consume water, unsweetened coffee, and or tea on fasting days. There is a modified version where you consume 25% of your calories on fasting days, which would amount to 400 to 600 calories for most people.

2. **The 5:2 Fasting Method** is consuming 25% of your normal caloric intake on two (non- consecutive) days per week. Some people will do a full 24-hour fast on one of their two fasting days, but that is not necessary unless you feel called to do so.

3. **Time-restricted fasting** is eating all your calories within an 8 or 10-hour window each day. Outside of that window, you would only have water, black coffee, and or unsweetened tea. Most people practice time-restricted fasting six days per week, with one day where you can eat throughout most of the day, but ideally sticking to just three meals with little to no snacking.

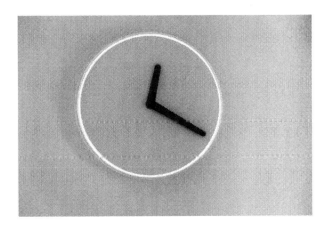

Say 'Good-bye' To Belly Fat

Aside from these three types of Intermittent Fasting, there is also the 3-Day water-only fast, which is self-explanatory, and the Fasting Mimicking Diet by Dr. Valter Longo of the Longevity Institute in Italy and California. The Fasting Mimicking Diet is based on five days. On day 1, you cut your calories in half (around 800 to 1,200 calories for most people if you eat 1,600 to 2,400 calories on a normal day). On days 2, 3, and 4, you eat 25 percent of your normal caloric intake (around 400 to 600 calories). On day 5, you go back to 50 percent, and on day six you are back to regular calories. Both of these more challenging fasts are usually done once per month. For people with more severe illnesses and cases of diabetes, it's recommended to do it more frequently, but always under professional supervision from your doctor.

What we've come to learn is that after about 18 hours of fasting, the process of cellular autophagy begins in which old, worn-out parts of cells are recycled into new and healthier parts. Cellular autophagy has been shown to slow the aging process, as well as lower the risk of cancer, heart disease, and neurodegeneration, while also boosting your immune system[18]. After about 24 hours there's an increase in this response, and after about 48 to 72 hours, there's a peak in cellular autophagy.

According to research at the Longevity Institute, which has been duplicated numerous times in various parts of the world, the fasting-mimicking diet, which is not a complete fast, since you still eat some calories on fasting days, has the same benefits as complete water-only fasting. It's shown to lower fasting glucose, blood pressure, cholesterol, and waist size especially for people with BMI over 30[19], as well as reduced risk of diabetes, heart disease, and cancer. It's even been shown to improve chemotherapy treatment.

Each of these fasts mentioned has shown to have significant health benefits, and a major one is improving insulin sensitivity and or reducing insulin resistance. That's why weight loss is also a key result or benefit from fasting. Additionally, fasting does not slow metabolism down like daily calorie restriction from traditional diets. Other health benefits include lowering blood pressure and cholesterol, improving gut health, and increasing HgH (human growth hormone), which is connected to fat loss, slowing the aging process, improving cognition, possibly reducing the risk of dementia, and possibly lowering the risk of certain cancers.

One surprising fact about fasting is that most people experience an energy boost on fasting days, or during their fasting window, as compared to non-fasting days. This could be due to the regulation of insulin as well as the increase in cognitive hormones. I can only suggest that you try a variety of these types of fasting to see which one suits your life and lifestyle the best. Any of them will help improve weight loss efforts by improving insulin sensitivity, gut health, and helping control calories.

ACTION PLAN SUMMARY to FASTING

Simply pick a type of fasting and try it for a week or two to see how you feel. Explore a variety of these and see which fasting works best for you.

Step 5

MOVE

Step 5: MOVE

How important is exercise? While it's true that 80 percent of your weight loss results come from your diet, research has shown again and again that one of the two most important things that you can do to impact your lifespan (length of life) and health-span (quality of life as you age) is exercise. Quitting smoking trades places with exercise for first or second place depending on the study. For example, being fit is associated with a 50 percent less chance of dying from heart disease. For middle-aged women that did little to no exercise (less than one hour per week), it increased their chance of early death by 52%, doubled their chances of cardiovascular disease, and increased their probability for cancer by 29% [20]. If you've been inactive and sedentary, simply by being active for one to three hours per week reduces your risk of chronic diseases and early death by 44 percent. That's HUGE!

The cool thing here is that it doesn't require going to a gym, spending hours each day on a dreaded treadmill and some funky exercise equipment, unless of course you like those things (which I happen to). You just need to stress your heart and lungs a bit, whether it's walking briskly, hiking, jogging, cycling, swimming, gardening, etc... and you need to challenge your muscles, bones, and joints several times per week by squatting, lifting, pulling, pushing, carrying, etc... and again- you don't need a gym membership. You can use your body weight, and maybe some dumbbells, exercise bands, or a few items around the house.

Say 'Good-bye' To Belly Fat

The Fitness Habit

Who you are today is basically a sum of your habits. And with all the marketing around fitness for the past 40 or so years, and still, only around ten to twenty-three percent of the population, depending on which study you look at, get the minimum recommended amount of exercise, so we know it's not a habit for most. Do you LOVE to exercise? If not, you're not alone, so don't beat yourself up with negative self-talk if you just don't enjoy it. But don't restrict exercise and being physically active to only going to the gym or doing long-distance running. There are countless ways to be physically active and get exercise in. I have a client that found mountain biking and kayaking later in life, and that's how he found fitness after decades of being sedentary and out of shape. I have a friend that after years of not exercising, started playing pickleball (one of the hottest trend these days along with frisbee golf) with friends and fell in love with it. She plays three days per week for two hours at a time. She's now added yoga to help maintain flexibility and balance.

Start thinking of physical activities you enjoyed as a kid or teenager— are there any you would like to revisit? Have you wanted to get back to playing basketball, beach volleyball, roller-skating, or rollerblading? Or how about activities that piqued your curiosity recently, but you haven't made it a priority to try? What about tennis, dance lessons, Zumba, or hiking? Maybe connect your fitness to a charity that has a strong meaning to you and sign up for an event like a 5K, 10K, or a triathlon? There are so many ways to become physically active and actually enjoy it. The key is to try things and find ones you enjoy, then turn them into HABIT.

Say 'Good-bye' To Belly Fat

Mindful Movement

Do the same with movement and exercise as you will be doing with 'Mindful Eating'. Pay attention to how your body feels during movement and exercise, and how it feels afterward. Notice muscles and joints as they push and pull your body— as they fatigue, and how they can push a little more if you truly desire more. Notice how your mind thinks and your mood changes with movement and exercise. That was my big "Ah-ha" moment that made the difference and helped me make exercise a habit. It's when I noticed that my anger and depression truly lifted, and my confidence and mood improved with exercise.

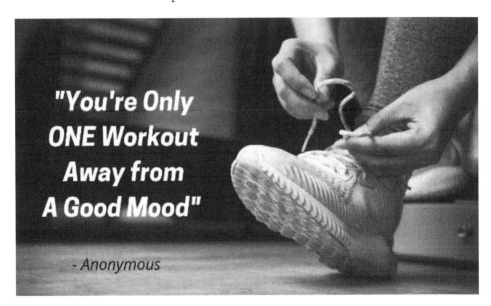

If you don't exercise at all, or you've been extremely inconsistent (you know, workout for 3 months—stop for 5 months—start again for 4 months— stop for 7 months—start again for 2 months—stop for 2 years), then I recommend focusing on consistency over anything else.

Say 'Good-bye' To Belly Fat

Don't try and do 45 minutes or hour-long workouts; instead, commit to six days per week and start with just 4 minutes (or longer if you wish, but commit to at least 4 minutes) of exercise twice per day, plus a 10-minute brisk walk. You can go longer, but commit to at least ten minutes. If the weather doesn't permit you to go outside for a walk, and you don't own a treadmill, you can march in place while moving your arms in all directions for 10 minutes while watching a television show or listening to a podcast.

Also, commit to getting your first session of exercise done early in the morning before you start the major items of your day. On top of added fat loss when exercising in a fasted state, there's truly no better way to start your day than accomplishing some self-care and getting a pump of endorphins. This will set you up for success and positive thinking far more than holding off till later and possibly getting too busy to even fit in 4 minutes of exercise (which you're truly never too busy; it's a lack of prioritization that may cause you to tell yourself that you are too busy to exercise for 4 minutes). I recommend drinking a full glass of water when you wake up, which kickstarts you towards your water goal as well, stretching for a minute or two, and then setting a timer on your phone or watch for 4 minutes (or longer), and get moving. Here's a sample 4-minute routine you might want to try:

- **30 seconds of planks (or upward dog to down dog)**
- **followed by 30 seconds of squats**
- **followed by 30 seconds of lying down leg raises**
- **followed by 30 seconds of jumping jacks...**

* You're halfway there at the 2-minute mark; repeat the four exercises for one more round and you've got your 4 minutes done!

Say 'Good-bye' To Belly Fat

At the end of the 4 minutes, ask yourself, 'do I feel better, same, or worse?' – 99 out of 100 times, you will feel better! You may feel so good that you want to do a few more minutes. That internal motivator is far more powerful for creating a habit and making this a lifestyle than following a fitness routine where someone told you to get 45 minutes of exercise. Which of these two are you more likely to quit, and which are you more likely to be willing to do for a long, long time?

Quick note— any additional minutes you do in your first exercise routine do NOT count towards your 2nd 4-minute routine because the principle here is that you are active multiple times throughout your day, so you identify as an active person, not the total minutes.

As you begin to make movement and exercise a habit, you will want to increase the amount of core exercises, plus increase the intensity by adding more weights and resistance and or doing some interval training. The key to long-term weight loss is to have a combination of building muscles along with exerting your cardiovascular system. You truly need both for long-term fat loss and health. Take a look at my *Get 4Ever Fit* Program

if you want a guided program to take you from any level, to being healthy, strong, flexible and fit in 90 days with 30 minutes or less per day, even if you are just starting out. There's a Free Month Bonus, so you actually get

Say 'Good-bye' To Belly Fat

ACTION PLAN SUMMARY to MOVE

Commit to moving every day. Identify where you are at today with your exercise level and where you need to start and how you can improve daily.

If you are sedentary, start with 4 minutes, two times per day, plus a 10-minute walk. Commit to this routine six days per week for the next three weeks.

If you exercise currently, but are not consistent, add in the 4 minutes twice per day as a minimum movement for days you do not do your regular workout or other physical activity.

Find ways you can exercise with a partner or as a family. It doesn't have to be formal exercise— it can be going for bicycle rides or hiking; it can be playing pickleball or tennis.

Build stronger muscles starting with body weight (push-ups, planks, squats, lunges, etc…) and then start using any form of resistance (exercise bands, dumbbells, barbells, exercise machines, household goods, etc…) Want a program that progresses you safely and effectively from any level to being strong, flexible, and fit in 30 minutes or less, check out my Get 4 Ever Fit program at www.get4everfit.com.

Say 'Good-bye' To Belly Fat

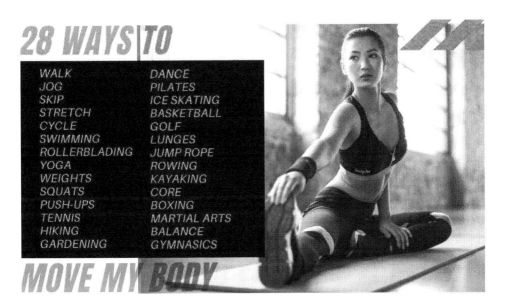

List 5 other ways that you like, or are curious to try, to move more and be physically active:

1. _____

2. _____

3. _____

4. _____

5. _____

Step 6

SLEEP

Say 'Good-bye' To Belly Fat

Step 6: SLEEP

Sleep is one of the most studied areas in health and wellness over the past 30 plus years. It's become such a hot topic since the research has clearly shown that sleep is directly connected to not only weight loss or weight gain, but also heart disease, diabetes, certain cancers, dementia, depression, and gut health. And according to a report by AAA based on dozens of studies involving car accidents, you are twice as likely to have a car accident if you sleep between 6 and 7 hours, instead of the normal 7.5 to 8.5 hours of sleep. If you get 5 to 6 hours of sleep, you are four times more likely to have an accident, and if you sleep 4 to 5 hours, you are 11 times more likely to have an accident[21]. Regardless of all the data and marketing to push for better sleep, most people still struggle to get good quantity or quality of sleep.

One of the main culprits is our electronics. Scrolling on social media, reading a book on a digital device (except this one if you are reading the eBook), working late on your computer, and watching television before bed, or even worse, while in your bed, have shown to significantly diminish your sleep quantity and quality. Why? First, the blue light from your screens tells your brain it's still daytime, so your body doesn't produce enough melatonin to help you fall asleep easily, much less stay asleep. One solution is blue-light blocking glasses, which have become very popular over the past few years. Also, certain devices have night-mode, where they shift to more red light and stop emitting blue light.

Say 'Good-bye' To Belly Fat

Aside from the blue light, there's also the content you're absorbing. Are you watching the news late at night? Or high-adrenaline, high-suspense shows? Are you caught up in other people's lives on social media and comparing your life to their magically perfect life? The content you're absorbing might be producing Cortisol, the stress hormone, which inhibits sleep. You may be thinking this is not an issue for you since you've been able to fall asleep to the television or after spending time on your phone in bed, which may be true— you're eventually crashing from exhaustion, but if you measure your sleep, you will notice more disruptions, plus less time in REM and deep state sleep, which are the keys to health and weight loss.

Another culprit that has been shown to negatively impact sleep is our diet. Sugar, caffeine, and processed foods disrupt our circadian rhythm and our gut health, both of which are tied to sleep. Again, you may be saying to yourself that you can have an espresso coffee at 10:00 pm at night, and still fall asleep by midnight. I am able to do that myself. The issue is that it disrupts our REM and deep state sleep. I use a Whoop Strap to measure my sleep, and it's loud and clear to me on how caffeine past 2:00 pm impacts my sleep quality, and often quantity as well. Most data suggest cutting caffeine out at least six hours, and ideally ten hours before bedtime, especially if you are sensitive to caffeine.

We've discussed how sugar and processed foods affect our "gut health"; and we've discussed how poor gut health affects our "sleep". We've turned to fast-food and processed foods for convenience, but at a heavy cost (pun intended) to not only our sleep but also our waistlines and our health.

Say 'Good-bye' To Belly Fat

Lack of exercise or being sedentary is also connected to poor sleep. As is having light in your bedroom at night whether it's from your electronics, an alarm clock, or a streetlamp outside your window-- all of which diminish sleep quality and often quantity. Blacking out your room is a quick and easy solution to help boost your sleep. Keeping your bedroom temperature at a cool 68 degrees (or cooler) is also key to helping you get a quality night's rest. When our body temperature rises if our bedroom is too warm, our heart rate increases, and we do not get into deeper states of sleep. Eating too close to bedtime will also increase your body temperature and negatively affect your sleep.

Lastly, I want to mention the power of napping, especially if you are not getting a high-quality 7 to 8.5 hour of sleep. There's so much research on the benefit of power naps that there are now books, Apps, audios, and gadgets to help you take a nap. The two key factors to napping are that you don't nap for too long, and don't nap too late. If napping causes you to struggle with sleep at night, then it might not be the best solution for you. You may also try 10 to 20-minute power naps and see if that refreshes you without affecting your sleep at night.

Most researchers suggest napping between 10 and 30 minutes is ideal for feeling refreshed, and between 30 and 90 minutes to help with reducing stress and anxiety[22]. Also napping between 1:00p and 3:00p seems to be the best time for most people, but it depends on your current sleep cycle and schedule. I know people that would go out to their car during their lunch break, take a 15 to 30 minute nap, and come back totally refreshed and upbeat for the afternoon part of their day.

Say 'Good-bye' To Belly Fat

Here are some steps to improve your sleep hygiene and get better quality and quantity of sleep.

ACTION PLAN SUMMARY to SLEEP

Stop drinking any caffeine at least 6 hours (ideally 10 hours) before bedtime

Stop eating at least two hours before bedtime. If you feel a little hungry, have herbal (chamomile) tea and see if that can curb your hunger. Chamomile helps with sleep.

Stop using electronics or watching television at least 45 to 60 minutes prior to going to bed, and don't go on your electronics or watch tv while in bed.

Exercise and move more— this will cause your body to sleep better as part of the exercise recovery processes

Listen to relaxing music, journal and or read a relaxing book, drink herbal tea. These are all ways to help you relax and get better sleep.

Blackout your room

Make sure your room temperature is a cool 64 to 68 degrees.

Say 'Good-bye' To Belly Fat

PUTTING IT ALL INTO PRACTICE

The most important factor in achieving your weight goals is *taking action* and putting this information into practice. There are several things you want to consider to get the most out of this information and make sure you are successful and your results are lasting— in essence, that you are turning these steps into habits and making this a lifestyle.

Accountability Partner

First and foremost, I HIGHLY recommend getting an accountability partner or partners. Research shows that having an accountability partner increases your chances of success by **600 percent**—that means you are 6X more likely to achieve your goals by having someone to help hold you accountable than if you go at this all alone. An accountability partner doesn't necessarily have to be doing this journey with you, but it helps and makes it more fun if they are also participating, and you are holding each other accountable. Consider even having a group of fiends, co-workers, or your family doing this together.

Choose Steps to Focus on First

Next, identify if you do better by focusing on two or three of the six steps, or by working on all six steps at once. Find what works best for you. There is no wrong answer- except choosing not to work any at all.

Say 'Good-bye' To Belly Fat

If you choose to work on two or three steps to start, be sure to really master them before moving to the others. You don't have to be perfect in any area, but feel confident that you are proficient. I love using the 85 percent rule. If you are making the better choices 85 percent of the time, you are proficient. If you are above 90 percent, you have mastered it.

I also suggest choosing one or two of the steps that you are struggling with the most, along with one that you are fairly successful in. Then identify the mindset, attitude, and habits around the area you are successful in, and see how you can transfer those to the step or steps you are struggling with the most. This is a great strategy to create major break-throughs.

Within each step, there are action items to work on which are critical to mastering that step as well as mastering your insulin and achieve lasting weight loss. There's a daily tracking sheet at the end of the book to help you track your progress each day, plus remind you of all the action items to work on.

Self-Awareness

It's important to know where you are today in each of these areas. You've heard it said before- It's hard to know where you are going, if you don't know where you currently are. Use the chart on the next page to rate your current habits or proficiency around the six steps on a scale of 1 (meaning poorly) and 7 (meaning excellent) for how well you feel you have these mastered.

Say 'Good-bye' To Belly Fat

The chart also lets you evaluate yourself at 1 month, 3 months, and 6 months, so you can get a better sense of your progress. Self-awareness is a key factor to making progress and avoiding wandering aimlessly which often ends in frustration and failure.

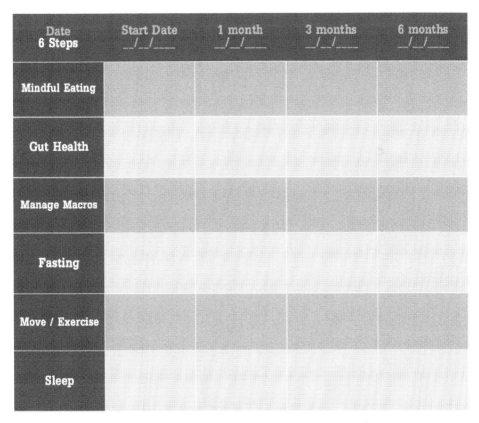

Rate your proficiency for each Step on a scale of 1 (poorly) to 7 (excellent)

Say 'Good-bye' To Belly Fat

Lastly, if you have a family, it important to get their support. Share your goals with them and your reason why this is important to you. Getting a spouse's support so you can schedule in things like exercise breaks or walks, or better yet- do some physical activities together. Get a commitment as a family to making some healthier food choices, or at least to put snacks and desserts in high cupboards, and only pulling them out once per week or every other week in order to support your journey. Whatever you feel you need to plan and get support, be proactive and ask for support. It's hard enough going at it alone, but it's 10X harder if your family or friends are doing everything to create more temptations or to sabotage your results.

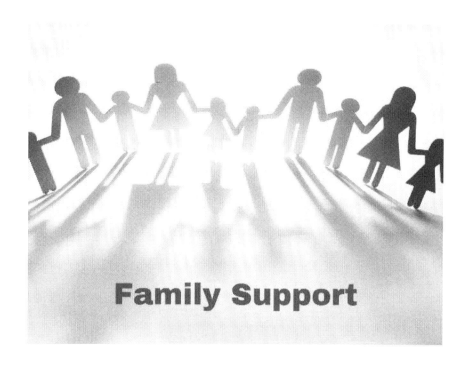

OVERCOMING OBSTACLES

With every new coaching client, I always ask, what are the top two obstacles they can foresee most likely to get in the way of their goals? If you can foresee them, then you can plan on how to respond without becoming overwhelmed, over-stressed, and frustrated, and end up quitting or giving up on your goals. There's always a solution. As Marie Forleo says, "Everything is Figure-outable".

Take a couple of minutes and identify two obstacles you will most likely encounter and could be the biggest challenges to hitting your weight loss goals and getting rid of belly fat. Write them down here, or in a separate journal. I do recommend having to journal daily during your weight loss journey to help you stay aware of your wins and challenges.

Most Probable Obstacles

1. _____

2. _____

Great, now spend a couple of minutes and truly connect to your highest and best self. How will you overcome each of these obstacles if and when they present themselves? Provide at least three ways in which you can and will respond to each obstacle if it presents itself.

Say 'Good-bye' To Belly Fat

Best Responses to Overcome Obstacle #1

1. _____

2. _____

3. _____

Best Responses to Overcome Obstacle #2

1. _____

2. _____

3. _____

FALLING OFF TRACK

I also want to mention that you are going to fall off track at times. It happens to every single person— and that's ok. I've been a health coach for twenty-five years and have coached thousands of clients. Trust me, not one person has been perfect. I've fallen off track continuously throughout my life and career, and I still do today. The key is to not have judgment about it. Don't beat yourself up and start a bunch of negative self-talk; that has never helped anyone. In fact, it most often makes things worse— far worse. Acknowledge and honor the fact that you noticed you fell

Say 'Good-bye' To Belly Fat

off track and want to get back on track. Instead of criticizing yourself or spending hours thinking about it, simply identify what one action you can do next to help get you back on track. Is it taking a few deep breaths and a walk in nature today? How about doing a few squats and planks while watching your favorite stand-up comedian or listening to your favorite music? Maybe it's drinking 80 ounces of water? Do any of these or any other healthy habit you can think of, and then go give yourself a 'high-five' in the mirror, as taught by the amazing Mel Robbins, in her book, *The High 5 Habit*. Remember, the goal is staying on track 85 or 90 percent of the time. This mindset alone will help you always stay near the tracks when you fall off, meaning you won't get too far off track and sabotage your results.

It's also important to know that you are exploring and learning about yourself throughout this process. You are exploring and learning about what your triggers are and how you can best respond to them; what foods serve you best, and which do not; what exercises or physical activities you enjoy, and which you dislike; how to get enough water each day; etc… Shifting your mindset from blame, guilt, and shame, over to curiosity, wonder, and exploration, will set you up for long-term success and a much more joyful journey.

FINAL THOUGHTS

I've decided to create a 7-Day Kickstart Program to help you jump-start your fat loss and your way to mastering your insulin. It includes a daily practice of exercise, water, meal plan, and even habits for good sleep hygiene. Download and print the 7-Day Jumpstart Program at https://myforeverfatloss.com.

Read through the 7 days and create your own grocery list, so you can be prepared. If there are foods you do not like, try your best to replace them with foods that have similar macros and that are from the same categories (fiber, polyphenols, prebiotics, probiotics, fiber, etc...). But don't stress about it either. Most importantly, go for real natural whole foods.

Also, pay attention to how you feel after each meal. Use the daily tracker, so you can track each day (print 1 copy for each day). This will help you notice which foods are working for you and which might be causing you inflammation of energy blockages. You will also be able to track the micro habits that comprise each of the six steps.

Losing belly fat is not as hard as you might be imagining, and it's more worth it than you might be imagining. Make the decision and follow through by putting these steps into practice. And remember, no one has ever regretted getting leaner, stronger, healthier and more fit.

Say 'Good-bye' To Belly Fat

Finally, know that being healthy, losing belly-fat, achieving health goals is not just for you. When you improve your health, you are impacting those around you, especially your family members and closest friends. Good health is contagious, so know that this is an important and noble cause. Stop sacrificing your health for those you love, and instead get healthy for those you love. You will have a far more positive impact on your life and theirs. Believe that it is not only possible, it is necessary.

I BELIEVE IN YOU.
NOW IT'S YOUR TURN TO BELIEVE IN YOU.

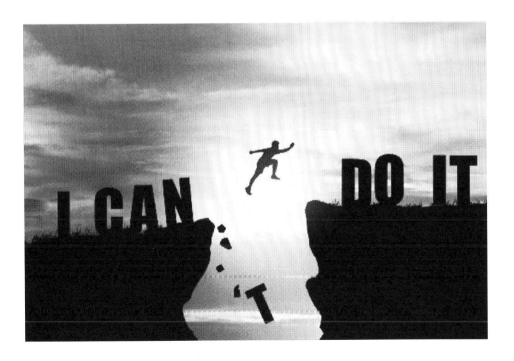

Say 'Good-bye' To Belly Fat

6 Steps to Mastering Your Insulin and Lasting Weight Loss

Daily Log Name: _____ Date: ___/___/_____

- **Mindful Eating:**
  Pre – during – post meal
  Breakfast ☐   Lunch ☐   Dinner ☐

- **Get Gut Healthy**
  ☐ Polyphenols
  ☐ Prebiotic Foods
  ☐ Probiotic Foods
  ☐ 30+ grams of fiber

- **Manage Your Macros:**
  ☐ Protein: 25-30%
  ☐ Carbs: 40-45%
  ☐ Fat: 25-30%
  ☐ Water: 80+ ounces

- **Fasting:** Type _____
  ☐ Fasting _____ hours / calories

- **Movement/Exercise:**
  2X 4+ minutes / 10+ minute walk)
  ☐   ☐   ☐

- **Rest / Sleep**
  ☐ 7.5 – 8.5 hours
  ☐ 10 – 45 min nap

Food/Drink (time) | Macro Nutrients | Reaction to Food

MEAL #1:
_____
Time: _____ am / pm

Calories:
Carbs:
Protein:
Fat:
Fiber:
Sugars:

☐ Energy Crash
☐ Bloating
☐ Food Cravings < 3 hours
☐ Irritability or mood dip
☐ Skin Irritation

MEAL #2:
_____
Time: _____ am / pm

Calories:
Carbs:
Protein:
Fat:
Fiber:
Sugars:

☐ Energy Crash
☐ Bloating
☐ Food Craving < 3 hours
☐ Irritability or mood dip
☐ Skin Irritation

MEAL #3:
_____
Time: _____ am / pm

Calories:
Carbs:
Protein:
Fat:
Fiber:
Sugars:

☐ Energy Crash
☐ Bloating
☐ Food Craving < 3 hours
☐ Irritability or mood dip
☐ Skin Irritation

SNACK:
_____
Time: _____ am / pm

Calories:
Carbs:
Protein:
Fat:
Fiber:
Sugars:

☐ Energy Crash
☐ Bloating
☐ Food Craving < 3 hours
☐ Irritability or mood dip
☐ Skin Irritation

TOTAL CALORIES: _____
Total PROTEIN: _____ g _____ %
Total CARBS: _____ g _____ %
Total FAT: _____ g _____ %
Total FIBER: _____ g _____ %

*Aim to stop eating at least 2 hours prior to bedtime

Polyphenols	Pre-biotic	Probiotic	Fiber	Sleep Hygiene
Artichoke	Artichoke	Cottage cheese	Apples	☐ No Caffeine 6+ hours prior to bedtime
Parsley	Apples	Kefir	Avocado	☐ No Food 2+ hours prior to bedtime
Strawberries	Asparagus	Kimchi	Beans	☐ Relax music, journal, book, and or tea before bed
Asparagus	Banana	Greek yogurt	Beets	☐ No Electronics or Television 1 hour prior to bedtime
Apples	Barley	Tempeh	Berries	☐ Room Temperature between 64 - 68 degrees F
Broccoli	Broccoli	Miso	Broccoli	☐ Blackout Room
Carrots	Cabbage	Sauerkraut	Bran	
Grapefruit	Cocoa	Kombucha tea	Coconut	
Black beans	Dandelion		Lentils	
Tofu	Garlic		Pears	
Flaxseeds	Jicama		Split peas	
Almonds	Leeks		Strawberries	
Walnuts	Mushroom		Sweet Potato	
Cinnamon	Oats		Whole grains	
	Onions		Flaxseed	
			Chia seeds	

For more guidance and help with your journey to better health, connect with me on social media at @vitalitybysergio on Facebook, Instagram, and LinkedIn.

Stay grateful, kind to yourself and others, and enjoy the journey.

Blessings,

Sergio